HOW I GOT
MY LIFE BACK

HOW I GOT
MY LIFE BACK

From
Granddad's Herbs
and
Food Medicine
Lessons

Joseph C. Okoye

Copyright © 2010 by Joseph C. Okoye.
Edited by: S.I. Okoye (Pharm. D)
Cover design by: Joseph C. Okoye

Library of Congress Control Number: 2010912909
ISBN: Hardcover   978-1-4535-6909-2
                 Softcover   978-1-4535-6905-4
                 Ebook   978-1-4535-6910-8

This book was printed in the United States of America.

To order additional copies of this book, contact:

Xlibris Corporation
1-888-795-4274
www.Xlibris.com
Orders@Xlibris.com
86238

Contents

Disclaimer

This book is a testimony. It does not in any way mean to substitute any treatment any individual is supposed to have with his or her health care professional. Always consult or discuss with your health care professional if you are on medication and intend to engage on any food therapy to check drug interactions with certain food plants you may take.

These statements have not been evaluated by the FDA or any other concerned food and drug administration and are not intended to diagnose, prevent, mitigate, treat or cure any diseases. The contents are based on the writer's exposure to a dear grandfather's lessons. A grandfather(herbalist) who treated many people and saved lives with natural food plants, the barks of certain trees, vegetables, fruits, seeds, plant roots, water, natural sea salts and certain types of fish. Individual results may vary depending on personal disposition.

This is a testimony of how I neglected my grandfather's herbs and food medicine lessons with the consequence of developing multiple health problems and how I got my life back by adopting my grandfather's wellness lessons on herbs and food medicine. The details of what I did to be healed and how I got my life back are discussed later in this book.

This is dedicated to my grandfather Stephen Dimel Okonkwo who in my youth had me around him during my school breaks. I learned a lot about his food habits, sickness prevention and natural healing by daily consumption of different types of plant foods as natural medicine(vegetables, fruits, fresh seeds, medicinal tree barks and plant roots), but did not adopt the values until later in my life;

To my parents Raymond Ekwonu and Maria Nwanyanwu Okoye who applied their acquired knowledge of plant medicines and techniques to treat my childhood illnesses;

To all people who help to prevent or minimize illnesses in the world

And Above all

To the Greater Glory of God, the Creator of all and the Sustainer of life by Whose inspiration I'm releasing this testimony for the good of all and to encourage people to focus on natural food plants for life in compliance with:

Geneses 1:29 **Then God said, "I give you every seed-bearing plant on the face of the whole earth and every tree that has fruit with seeds in it. They will be yours for food."**

Exodus 23:25 **"Worship the LORD your God, and his blessing will be on your food and water. I will take away sickness from among you,"**

Ezek. 4:9 **"Now take some wheat, barley, beans, peas, millet and spelt, mix them all together an make bread"**

Biography of my Grandfather

My Grandfather Stephen Dimel Okonkwo was born in 1865 in Enugwu-Ukwu, East Nigeria West Africa. He passed on at the age of 105. The city where he worked in his early life had many traditional herbalists in the community and he learned a lot from them on how to treat with herbs (plant roots, nuts, fruits, tree bark and certain plant roots). He learned the importance of feeding the body with naturally unprocessed vegetables, fruits and nuts with selected fish like salmon and a little dried meat. He used the sun to dry foods required for long storage.

He lived a very healthy life and had never been to any hospital in his life time. He treated many people and saved many lives including a young man whose ill health defied a hospital treatment and was discharged by a medical doctor to stay home and die. My grandfather's plant food medicine revived him and he came back to life.

My grandfather acquired from his early mentor the plant type used for treating poisonous snake bites. His mentor was passionately searching for herbs in the forest for treatment of different diseases. He said one day his mentor sighted a monkey jumping from a tree branch to a tree branch. The monkey jumped onto a branch where a dangerous snake had stretched its self resting. Instantly the snake bit the monkey. The monkey jumped away from the snake, diverted to another tree and kept on jumping from tree to tree.

He curiously observed the monkey's reaction. The monkey got to a particular tree and stopped. It plucked the leaves of this plant, Chewed into a paste, rubbed on the snake bite on its body and ate some of the leaves. His mentor having observed what the monkey did went and marked that particular tree as one of the plants for treating snake bites. He said his mentor used the leaves of that particular plant type to treat people bitten by snakes. My grandfather learned that from him. He also learned from his mentor that animals like goats which are reared as domestic animals in some cultures of the world were used to identify plants for human consumption.

Prologue

What led to the writing of this Book?

It is about prolonged negligence of natural preventive and curative food remedies within my reach and the resulting adverse consequences on my health. It is about my late adoption of unprocessed food plants resulting to my cure of multiple illnesses which I suffered for six years. I completely regained my good health. I felt that my body healed itself with the aid of the natural food plants.

The natural way human beings were meant to nourish and sustain the bodies were already contained in the word of God, The Old Testament Bible. We humans are endowed with the free will to choose what we want. The choices we make in what we eat and drink contribute to our wellness or ill health. Organic foods and unprocessed natural drinks are more amenable to living organisms like our bodies than chemical or synthetic substances.

Our Creator has already set forth for His created beings the right foods to eat to be healthy. Human bodies are more disposed to natural food plants (vegetables, fruits, seeds /nuts) than artificially processed foods with ingredients/chemicals foreign to the human bodies.

My Grandfather relied on herbs and food medicines for healthy living. He used sea salts in his foods and for its multiple natural remedies. He carefully avoided processed salts. Greater percentage of people who had no access to natural sea salts for a long time developed different types of **thyroid** problems linked to lack of iodine which is abundantly available in sea salts and sea weeds in the natural form.

My Grand father's lessons focused on giving the body the natural foods the body needed to maintain good health. He consumed more alkalizing foods and less acidifying foods all the time (see p.51 D-E). He never went to any conventional hospital yet he lived 105 years before he passed away.

The purpose of this book is to expose the consequences of my negligence of the natural foods in total preference to unnatural or artificially processed foods which resulted to my multiple illnesses and how I got my life back. My health recovery started from the memories of my early childhood observances of my Grandfather's food habits; and the natural healing he administered to different people with health problems including me. It will further expose how total change of my diet sucked out all my ill health from my body within six weeks.

Some may take less or more time depending on individual's stage of health condition, personal discipline and determination. I'm now in control of what I eat and what I don't eat. It is not what my body wants or feels like wanting but rather the right thing I decide to give to my body. Control and discipline is the key to the right choices of what we give to our bodies.

CHAPTER 1

How I Got My Life Back:

I earlier mentioned my negligence of the natural foods in total preference to unnatural or artificially processed foods which resulted to my multiple ill-health. In my early life as a child, I remember that I avoided eating vegetables. I had a limited choice for few types of fruits and nuts available to me. There were many types of fruits which I did not like to eat. I could not explain why I hated eating vegetables and variety of fruits; but I remembered that my mother provided them for me to eat but for what I could not understand, I did not like eating vegetables at all and I had taste for very few fruits.

I remembered that my mother provided alternate meals void of vegetables whenever I refused to eat meals containing vegetables. The habit continued even when I was around my Grandfather during my secondary school break periods. I observed that my Grandfather was always eating lots of vegetables, fruits with dried meat and fish. I disliked what he was eating and whenever I was offered any food containing vegetables, I would finish the rest of the meal except vegetables in the meal. Even after I got married, I still had problems eating vegetables and whenever I tried to eat vegetables, it was a very small quantity each time. The fruits I had a taste for were very few. I did not realize what I was missing and the later consequence on my health. My taste buds favored processed foods more.

I later realized that in my early childhood, I was not challenged to take vegetables as part of my meals whether I liked it or not. My refusal to take vegetables was allowed instead of making it mandatory. I was allowed to get away with my not liking vegetables. The first problems I had were anemia, kidney stones and my immune system was always compromised. I was sick a lot of times in my childhood.

In late 2002, I relocated to the United States and a year after my arrival, **I had multiple problems ranging from kidney stones, tendonitis, prostrate problem, pneumonia, shoulder joint problems, hyperglycemia, pains at the corner of my ascending and transverse colon, eye problem (blurred vision and dryness)**

The first prescription drug I had for my prostrate had some adverse side effects on my body. My lungs cells were collapsing resulting to my breathing problems. I discontinued and resorted to natural food supplements. In my subsequent prescription I was given a different type of drug. My body could not accommodate the side effects, dizziness and drowsiness which were very frustrating. I resorted to drinking much coffee to counter the side effect of drowsiness. I still continued with my old habit of consuming more processed foods without checking the ingredients my body was reacting to.

In the later part of 2007 and early 2008, I was contemplating on going for a colonoscopy to check if I was developing colon cancer. I had no health insurance and when I called a hospital to check what it would cost me since I had no health insurance and the pains were getting severe, I was told $1,800. This coincided with the time I was looking for an herbal store to purchase supplements for my wife. I ran into a herbal store where the owner helped to find the supplements I was looking for.

I found the owner of the herbal store Dr. Kwaku A. Appau (N.D) to be very knowledgeable. We talked a lot about nature's foods and their benefits to the body. I talked about my late grandfather's eating habits. I talked about how knowledgeable my grandfather was about herbs and how my grandfather treated and brought back to life a young man who was discharged from a hospital and declared by a doctor that he would die because there was no hope of the young man's survival. His ill health defied all hospital drugs.

I told him how my grandfather went to the forest and collected different plant leaves and roots, tree barks and some seeds which he cut and pounded in a mortar with pestle. The concoction was mixed with water and administered to the young man. Shortly after he ingested the concoction, it was noticed that he was responding to the treatment. He took the mix for some more days and recovered his health completely. This was a patient already declared to die by a medical doctor. A lot of times, natural approach to treatment saves lives.

Getting back, my life started after narrating the above story to the herbal store owner; thereafter the entire memory of what I observed my grandfather eating when I was young came back to me. I remembered my grandfather was very strong as an old man and he lived *105* years before he passed on and he never went to any hospital in his life. His immediate younger sister who adopted same principle lived *110* years. My grandfather knew a lot about different plants and seeds used to cure diseases. I asked myself. "WHY CAN'T I JUST TRY THIS?"

I instantly took a decision to eat everything I observed my Grandfather eating when I was growing up. I still was not able to quickly adjust to a new diet until early October 2008. The first thing I did one day was to pack all the processed, packaged and canned foods and put them out of my sight. I went to the farmer's market in my neighborhood and bought variety of vegetables and fruits, unripe plantain which my grandfather was eating a lot of with vegetables, red palm oil and other fruits and nuts.

I tried different recipes at different times and was able to develop palatable recipes out of vegetables, fruits, fresh nuts and fish. I avoided meat for some time and later was including it in very small quantities once in a while; but only none-hormone, none anti-biotic treated meat and fish (especially omega-3-rich sardine, salmon, herring, Mackerel and tuna etc). Vegetables, fruits and nuts for protein were enough.

The good news was that six weeks from the time I changed my diet, all the multiple health problems I had completely disappeared from my body. I noticed a big change in my health. I lost 21 pounds within the period of 6 weeks. My blurred vision resolved, I noticed clearer and sharper memory, increased energy, my abdominal pains stopped. I started sharing my testimony about "How I got my life back" to relatives and friends around me.

I learned that **illness prevention** is an individual's responsibility. It is easily accomplished with natural plants as food. Illness prevention is better and cheaper than cure. It gives joy and makes one feel in control of one's health. The details of all I did to get my life back are explained in the subsequent chapters. I combined different vegetables, fruits and nuts, according to what they are believed to prevent and heal and the results were excellent. Food plants have become my health corner stone which I neglected for a very long time.

CHAPTER 2

The Natural Regimen
That Brought My Life Back:

Having done away with my past eating habits and menus which consisted of processed acidifying foods and drinks, the next thing I did was to list all the food plants and herbs I observed my Grandfather eat and the herbs he used. Some were equivalent substitutes which he often used for himself; administered to me and other people with different health problems.

Among the leaves he got freely from the close by woods and forests do have substitutes in the international or local natural food markets. Parts of the world have different species of plant fruits, herbs and vegetables but the nutrients are the same in some and slight variations in others. Some have specific healing and **nutritive** values that deal specifically with certain ill health; while others have **supportive** nutrients.

The important thing is to get a variety of natural plant foods available in your environment; Sort them according to what you want to achieve. Plan palatable menus for yourself and strictly follow your regimen. Occasionally check the PH of your body with the use of the pH testing paper available in natural supplement stores or online. If the pH of your body indicates more acidic, reduce the acidifying foods you are consuming and increase vegetables and fruits ingestion to adequately alkalize your body. What I have written here is what I strictly followed to get my life back and I strongly believe that any one who adopts my regimen in its entirety would surely experience a change in his or her health.

Breakfast:
Banana 1
Radishes 4
Pineapple 6 small pieces
Dates 6
Strawberry or other types of berries 5
Grapes (with the seeds) 6
Peanuts (30 pieces)
All except dates are cut or sliced in small bits and sprinkled with peanuts

Tea beverages: Varied natural herb tea and Ginger (ground), Lemon, Lime, Turmeric & radishes (all grounded with the peels)
Honey 1tbsp

Breakfast (alternate menu-1):
Avocado 1 and sea salt
Seeded grapes 6
Pineapple 6 small pieces
Banana 1, peanuts 30 pieces
Radishes 4, strawberry 4
Red apple 1(seeds are eaten separately towards cancer prevention) Walnuts and (or) peanuts or almonds 30 pieces (without additives are healthful) and **Tea as above.**

Breakfast (alternate menu-2):
Apple 1
Banana 1
Grape seeds 6
Peanuts 30 pieces

Other menus for breakfast or snacks in between meals
(according to desired taste):

Avocado cream with nuts:
Pureed avocado with sea salt
Crushed pineapple
Shredded ginger
Radishes
Coconut
Mixed nuts (walnuts and peanuts)

Banana snack:
Sliced banana 1, Ginger, Sliced coconut and (peanuts, walnuts).

Avocado juice:
Crushed avocado, sea salt, purified water and honey

Lunch:
High fiber Whole grain Spaghetti (1/2 cup boiled)
Mixed vegetable sauce(ginger, garlic, lemon, Dates, lime, bell pepper, hot pepper, carrot, broccoli, spinach, turmeric, beet leaves, lettuce, onions, sea salt, cucumber and red palm oil) ½ cup, Green vegetables (collard green, turnip green) 1 cup, Banana 1 or pineapple ½ cup, beets 6 slices, and Dates 6.

Lunch:
Chopped Avocado 1, salmon,
Mixed vegetable sauce ½ cup
(ginger, garlic, lemon, Dates, lime, bell pepper, hot pepper, carrot, broccoli, spinach, turmeric, beet leaves, lettuce, Red onions, sea salt, cucumber and red palm oil) Green vegetables (collard green, turnip green) 1 cup
Banana 1 or pineapple ½

Lunch:

Boiled unripe plantain, Red palm oil, Vegetables (turnip green & collard green), Mixed vegetable sauce (ginger, garlic, lemon, lime, bell pepper, hot pepper, carrot, broccoli, spinach, lettuce, red onions, sea salt, cucumber and red palm oil (for nutrients and preservation).

Lunch (alternate-1):

Beans portage with plantain and salmon (size 2/3 cup cooked), Banana 1, Vegetables (collard green, turnip green, and parsley), Mixed vegetable sauce (as described above)

Lunch (alternate-2):

Avocado 1, Brown beans 2/3 cup cooked
Vegetables(selection or combination of collard green, turnip green, mustard green, kale) Tea (with Lemon, Lime, ginger, Turmeric & radishes—all grounded with the peels) Honey

Dinner:

Red cabbage (slightly boiled) with coconut oil spread, avocado and sea salt, hot tea with (ginger, Lemon, Lime, Turmeric, radishes (all grounded with the peels) and Honey

Dinner (alternate-1):

Cooked mashed unripe plantain 1 Soup with mixed vegetable concoction (occasionally with fish and locally raised reduced fat goat meat-free of injected synthetic hormones).

Dinner (alternate-2):

Avocado 2 and sea salt, Banana 1, dates 5, blanched green vegetables—1 cup, mixed vegetable sauce (ingredients as above), Pineapple 6 (small pieces), Mixed nuts (wall nuts, cashew, pecan, peanuts) & **Hot tea** with (Ginger, Lemon, Lime, Turmeric & radishes (all grounded with the peels), Honey.

Dinner (alternate-3):

Beans portage with unripe plantain, sea salt, dried fish, dried crayfish or shrimp, pepper and palm oil, (2/3 cup), Vegetables (selection or combination of collard green, turnip green, mustard green, kale), Mixed vegetable concoction (ginger, garlic, lemon, lime, bell pepper, hot pepper, carrot, broccoli, spinach, lettuce, red onions, sea salt, cucumber and palm oil—for nutrients and preservation).

Dinner (alternate 4)

Raw broccoli, red cabbage, green cabbage, carrot, bell pepper, none-monosodium-glutamate-ingredient salad dressing and fish(salmon, sardine mackerel, or other types with high omega-3)

Other general precautions I adopted towards getting my life back:

I had to read the ingredients on the packet of any food from the grocery and avoided eating any food with the following ingredients: Mono sodium glutamate, partially hydrogenated oil, talc, aluminum, food colors and carrageen an.

I avoided drinking pops, sodas, tonics sweetened with sugar—(to avoid weight gain) and aspartame to avoid ill health. I used Stevia plant sweetener. I avoided processed foods for the unknown degree of heat during processing which could result to likely presence of burnt or overheated and denatured food which can lead to carcinogens and hence ill health like cancer which is almost endemic in civilized parts of the world. I avoided warming foods in **plastic containers** in the microwave to avoid any danger of leaching plastic chemicals into the food. I avoided cow milk and cow meat suspected to be injected with **synthetic hormones.**

Water:

The importance of drinking sufficient clean water daily can not be overemphasized. It is a must to avoid health problems. I drink not less than 64 oz of filtered water daily.

Images of Sample Menus that Brought my Life Back

Tea

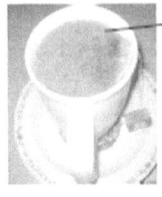

Any choice herb tea, water, crushed ginger, radishes, turmeric, lemon and lime; 1 1/2 minutes heating in microwave. Honey added occasionally.

Fruit breakfast

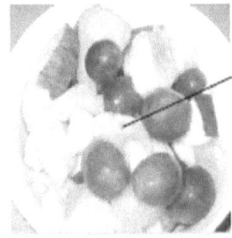

Banana, grapes with seeds, apple/seeds, pinaple, and cocktail peanuts (without additives)

Lunch

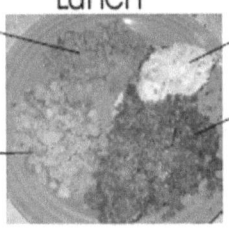

Mixed vegetable sauce(ginger, garlic, lime, lemon, bell pepper, hot pepper, carrots, broccli, turmeric, beet leaves, lettuce, red onions, sea salt cucumber and red palm oil).

Boiled brown Beans portage with unripe plantain, dried crayfish/shrimp, pepper, sea salt, red palm oil and dried fish.

Salmon fish

Blanched green vegetables (Collard green, turnip green) OR: (Mustard green, Kale as alternate choice) and sea salts, ground dry crayfish/shrimp

Dinner & Tea as above

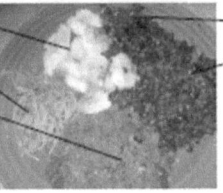

Banana

whole grain high fiber Spaghetti

Mixed vegetable sauce(ginger, garlic, lime, lemon, bell pepper, hot pepper, carrots, broccli, turmeric, beet leaves, lettuce, red onions, sea salt cucumber and red palm oil).

Dates

Blanched green vegetables (Collard green, turnip green) OR: (Mustard green, Kale as alternate choice) and sea salts, ground dry crayfish/shrimp

Alternate Dinner & Tea as above

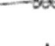

Mixed vegetable sauce(as Above)

whole grain high fiber Spaghetti

Dates

Beets

Apple with seeds

Blanched green vegetables (Collard green, turnip green) OR: (Mustard green, Kale as alternate choice), sea salts, and ground dry crayfish or shrimp.

CHAPTER 3

Preparation of Mixed Vegetable Sauce (concoction)

(i) Wash thoroughly and crush a bunch each of broccoli, lettuce, beet leaves, plus 20 balls of lemon, 20 balls of lime, 3 balls of red onion, 6 bell pepper, 3 cups of fresh hot pepper (before grinding), 2 cucumbers, 3 cups of red palm oil, 4 cups of fresh turmeric roots, 6 fresh carrots, 10 ginger roots, 50 balls of garlic and unprocessed natural sea salts to taste.

(ii) Put all in a covered pot and heat at low temperature; the red palm oil heats up fast, watch and turn off heat before the red palm oil starts to boil (the heat should be equivalent to the blanching heat). Do not allow boiling. Mix the concoction and taste to make sure you have enough sea salt. Move the pot away from the hot burner and allow to cool, putting away the quantity to be used within few days in the refrigerator and others in the freezer.

Note: The initial low heat is to avoid overheating in the subsequent future warming up. USES: The mixed vegetable sauce or concoction can be used on any choice menu and be taken twice daily.

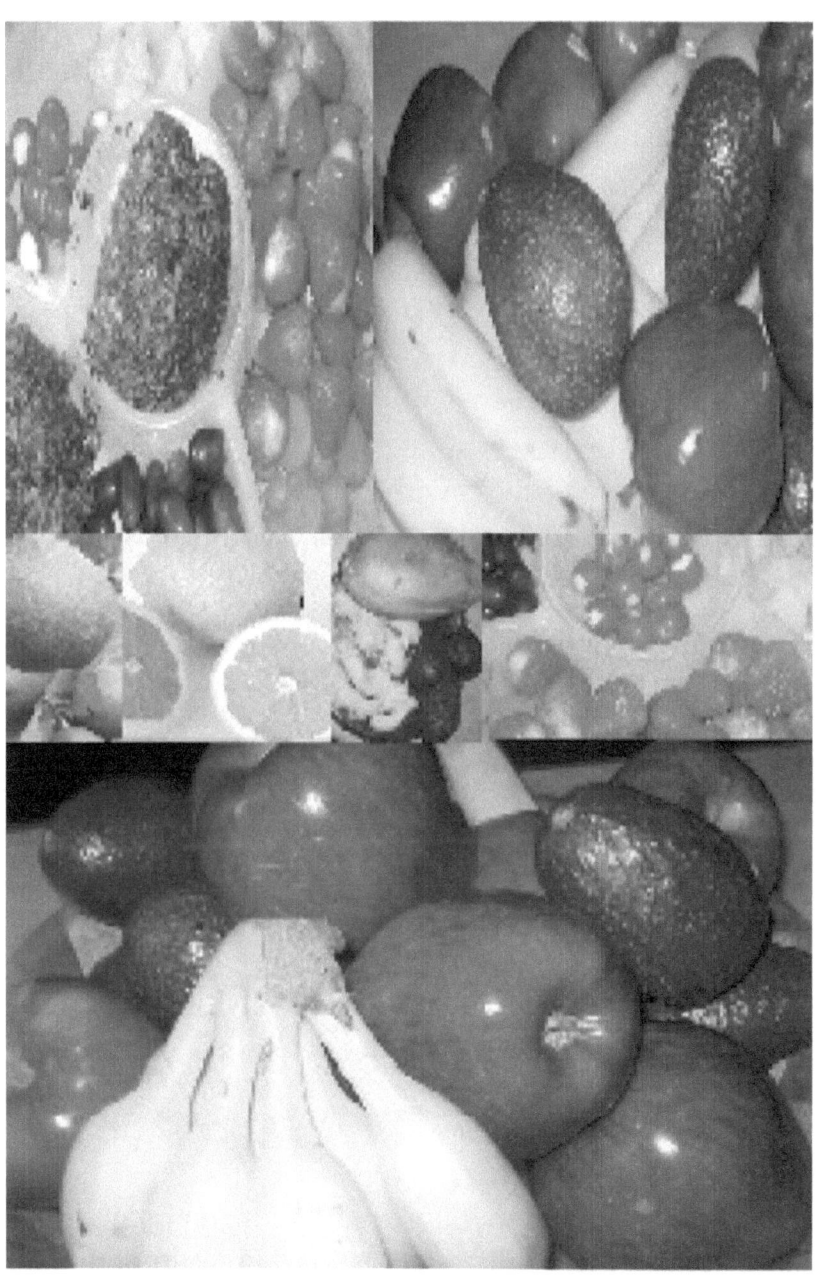

**Images of Sample Food Plants
That Brought My Life Back**

CHAPTER 4

Why I Chose My Regimen:

The first reason was to subject my body to food plants that support and prevent illness with hope and in line with:

Geneses 1:29 Then God said, "I give you every seed-bearing plant on the face of the whole earth and every tree that has fruit with seeds in it. They will be yours for food."

Exodus 23:25 "Worship the LORD your God, and his blessing will be on your food and water. I will take away sickness from among you".

I believed before trying and I believed more when I experienced a positive result leading to my testimony. There are values in food plants leading to diseases prevention and cures.

Food plants, Drinks and Believed Remedies:

Clean drinking Water:

Body hydration and temperature regulation, maintains healthy brain, increases metabolism and helps weight loss, maintains skin and helps reduce wrinkles, cleanses the system and helps prevent kidney stones.

Food Plants, Drinks, Believed Prevention & Remedies Continued:

Grapes with seeds:
Powerful antioxidant, cancer, leukemia and tumor

Apricot:
Anemia, tuberculosis, asthma, bronchitis, and blood poisoning by toxin,

Orange:
Asthma, bronchitis, tuberculosis, pneumonia, rheumatism, kidney stones, cholesterol, diabetes, arthritis, high blood pressure, helps alcohol addicts to withdraw from alcohol, reduces outpouring of mucus secretions from sinuses.

Garlic:
Lowers cholesterol; Anti bacterial and antiviral, cancer and tumors prevention, decongestant, lowers Blood pressure, antifungal, improves blood circulation.

Okra:
Blood sugar absorption regulation, prevents constipation, gas, laxative, promotes good bacteria, boiled slimy okra with lemon revitalizes hair, heals ulcer.

Celery:
Lowers blood pressure, arthritis remedy, rheumatic disease remedy, anti-inflammatory to swollen glands, appetite suppression (weight loss)

Cabbage:
Remedies for: Anti inflammation, cancer, ulcer, headache, asthma, bronchitis and other digestion problems, gastritis (inflammation of the lining of the stomach).

Carrot:
Antiseptic, promotes healthy skin, hair and nails. Promotes bone health, eye health, blood cleansing and building properties, cancer prevention and remedy, heart health, promotes healing of wounds, cuts and resolves inflammation; Blood pressure and lowering of cholesterol, menses regulation; anti colitis (colon inflammation), weight loss, urinary health, kidney and liver cleansing, gall bladder health, Alzheimer, diuretic, dispels phlegm / mucus in the throat, prevents baby jaundice in the womb, promotes fertility, lowers blood sugar.

Cucumber:
Diuretic, cleansing, gout, arthritis and tapeworm, eczema, skin health

Peanuts:
Cancer prevention, diabetes, and coronary heart diseases

Apples:
Teeth, gum, cholesterol, constipation, digestion, gout, rheumatism, anti virus,

Grapefruits:
Appetite inhibitor (weight loss), nerve health, arthritis, helps to remove worms (by the seeds), skin health improvement.

Honey:
Heals wounds, anti fungal, anti bacterial, asthma, cold (with ginger and lemon), cleanses blood.

Lemon:

Blood cleanser, antiseptic, use on wounds, heart health(potassium), sting pain reliever, gall stone, kidney stone, Diuretic, calms and improves stomach function, Insect repellant, the peel treats Colic (stomach pains or spasm), relieves pains of varicose veins, inflammation of veins, and improves circulation to a higher degree, preserves food, resolves acne and eczema and improves skin tone.

Red Onions:

Anti cancer, improves blood circulation, normalizes cholesterol, antibiotic, astringent for insect bite in combination with sea salt.

Ginger:

Anti nausea, anti diarrhea (with sea salt), menstrual cramps relief, cold relief, eases headaches, cancer/tumor growth, aides digestion.

Cauliflower:

Promotes healthy cholesterol, prevents cancer, heart health,

Banana:

Energy booster, heals ulcers, burns, gout, wounds, constipation, treats diarrhea (with sea salt), arthritis, anemia and constipation. Anti wrinkle (leave mashed banana on the face for 30 minutes, wash with warm and cold water respectively),heartburn, wart treatment, prevents cramps, intestinal disorders, kidney stones, arthritis, allergies, urinary disorders, tuberculosis bacteria (with stem extract), mosquito bite, treats poison ivy and rashes, boiled banana flower liquid decreases menstrual bleeding, burnt banana leaves relieves hiccup.

Unripe Plantain:

Diabetes (Unripe plantain has less sugar and more starch; while ripped has more sugar and less starch). Ripened plantain has the same support as ripened banana.

Coconut:

Weight loss (it boosts metabolism),aids digestion, heart health, lowering of cholesterol, helps rid off viruses, reduces cancer risk, controls diabetes, anti-aging.

Walnuts:

Heart health, lowers cholesterol.

Strawberry:

Prevents cancer, aids weight loss. Gum health and tartar reducer from teeth.

Radishes:

Liver disorder, gall bladder stone, Cancer.

Broccoli: Powerful anti cancer,
Side effect: gas (can be controlled with ginger and or garlic)

Lettuce: Nerve health, reproductive health,

Hot Pepper: Prevents liver disease, Obesity (aids weight loss), Constipation relief, Arthritis relief, anti cancer, Anti aging, asthma relief, kills ulcer bacteria, reduces bad cholesterol and triglyceride.

Dates: laxative, energy giver, provides relief for alcoholic intoxication, repairs cells, heart health.

Collard green: Anti cancer, heart health, nerve health, weight loss.

Kale: Helps digestion, cancer, major source of fiber, eye health, anti cataract, anti aging, joint problems.

Mustard green: For diabetes: low calories, anti cancer, heart health, bone health

Turnip Greens: Rheumatoid arthritis relief, promotes colon health, reduces risk of colon cancer, atherosclerosis, promotes lung health, nerve health.

Pineapple: Regulates gland (goiter), useful for digestive disorder, Bronchitis, excess mucous, stuffy nose, High blood pressure, Arthritis. Aids in removal of intestinal worms, alleviates diphtheria, sore throat, nausea, and constipation.

Lime:
Use for sore throat (with honey), relieves irritation of mosquito bite, protects eyes from degeneration, relieves headaches, fever; anti rheumatic, antiseptic, antiviral, cold relief, helps memory, Intestinal problems, jaundice, high blood pressure, diarrhea, dysentery, pile, indigestion, bad breath, dandruff and acne. Great for skin care, Shrinks pores, complexion enhancer(with cucumber), removes dead skin & odors; cleaning, air fresheners, Removal of deposits, eczema, **It can be consumed orally and or applied directly to the skin.**

Papaya (Pawpaw):
Digestion, Constipation, anti aging, infections of the colon and can help break down pus and mucus. Cancer, nausea, Diarrhea, raw juice for skin problems, juice with honey alleviates tonsil.

Crushed seeds and honey expels worms, helps to treat piles and chronic diarrhea; Juice applied to swelling prevents pus formation, applied to warts, pimples, corns, horn, or abnormal outgrowth of the skin and other skin diseases, juice removes freckles or brown spots from the skin. A paste of the seeds applied on the skin treats ringworm. Slices of green fruits rubbed over meat and boiled makes the meat tender.

Menstrual disorder: Unripe papaya aids contraction of the uterus and promotes proper menstrual flow.

Cirrhosis of the liver:
Seeds (alleviate cirrhosis of the liver caused by alcoholism, malnutrition, drug etc; a tablespoonful of grinded seeds, and crushed lime with the peel three times daily for a month), dysentery (treated with pawpaw latex and seeds).

Juice of raw papaya with honey can be applied over inflamed tonsils, diphtheria and other throat disorders, Prevents and reduces infection,

Spleen enlargement:
Peeled pawpaw soaked in vinegar or peeled raw pawpaw with pepper treats spleen enlargement caused by malaria, also ripe papaya

Leaf Pulp: prevents blood loss from wound and promotes healing. Leaf extract is purgative and induces birth, treats hernia and mucous urethra or inflammation, reproductive organs caused by infection, alleviates painless ulceration formed during the primary stage of syphilis.

Fresh latex: is smeared on boils, warts and freckles,

Bad effect:

Causes expulsion of embryo. Do not use during pregnancy.
—application to whitlow helps it to burst
—pawpaw root with salt or crushed seeds induce birth

Pawpaw leaf tea and fruit: contains a substance that dissolves surface cell debris making it a great facial peel.
—used for treatment of malaria

Crushed leaves are used externally to reduce headaches and cuts.

The stem sap treats fungal diseases e.g. ringworm.

Juice from the fruit is used to treat skin infections, cuts and ringworm. Liquid pressed from the plant and fruit is taken to remedy intestinal parasites and stomach ache.

—root is crushed to produce a juice, which is applied directly to ringworm.

—unripe pawpaw with unripe pineapple, lime, helps to treat malaria,

—latex from unripe fruit or trunk is used to treat eczema, razor bumps.

Beets:
Constipation, gout, kidney problem, leukemia, tumor/cancer, heart health, blood pressure, varicose veins, blood builder and cleanser, liver health, gall bladder, bile duct, menstrual problem, dysentery, tooth aches, skin problem, headache.

Palm Oil:
Increases the good HDL cholesterol levels, heart health

Watermelon:
Heart health, prevents cancer, alleviates male reproductive dysfunction

Turmeric:
Aids digestion, liver detoxifier, relieves arthritis pain, regulates menstruation, improves memory and prevents Alzheimer, increases metabolism and weight loss. Turmeric applied to the skin treats eczema and heals wounds, also relieves heartburn, stomach ulcers, and gallstones. Reduces inflammation, prevents /supports treatment of cancer, pain killer, arthritis, rheumatoid, turmeric is good as food and fabric dye.

Pomegranate:
Helps prevent hardening of the arteries (atherosclerosis), juice reduces incidence of heart attack, stroke, cholesterol, stress, Pomegranate contains high antioxidants, blood thinner, promotes blood flow, reduces arteriosclerosis, promotes good cholesterol and lowers bad cholesterol, reduces incidence of breast and skin cancer, Prevents prostate cancer, osteoarthritis, protects against cartilage damage, the seeds are good for the colon, provides anti-inflammatory substances.

Sea Salt:
Sea salt contains iodine and many other minerals, enhances natural healing, **stabilizes irregular heartbeats**, regulates blood pressure with water, **extracts excess acidity from the body, balances sugar levels in the blood**; reduces diabetes, promotes **nerve cells health and transmitters, promotes absorption of food** through the intestine. **Clears the lungs of mucus;** catarrh, sinus congestion, **muscle cramps prevention,** Protects body

from diseases, it prevents ear infection, treats eczema, removes dead skin, prevents dizziness, exhaustion and convulsions, helps energy level, regulates metabolism, prevents gout, varicose vein, promotes nerve cells' communication and regulates sleep.

Varied selection of fruits and vegetables:

I had varied selection of fruits and vegetables from the under listed titled:[Sickness Prevention and Natural Healing with Herbs and Food Medicine]. **They have been my source of good health till date.**

CHAPTER 5

Sickness Prevention and Natural Healing with Herbs and Food Medicine:

Cholesterol Normalization, Reduction of Homocysteine (amino acid from the by product of meat consumption), anti-aging, heart health:

Lemon, cinnamon, garlic, lemon-grass, beets, bee honey, okra, acai berry(heart health, cholesterol),apple, Red onion, oats, cauliflower, bitter kola, grape& seeds, soy, coconut, walnuts, strawberry, broccoli(with honey,& ginger) kiwi, turnip green, romaine lettuce, endive, sea weeds, water melon, oranges, cantaloupe, palm oil, pepper, sesame, sunflower, hibiscus flower, pomegranate (atherosclerosis and heart attack prevention), Dates, tangerine (cholesterol), avocado(anti-aging, heart health stroke, cholesterol), cranberry, salmon(omega3), sea salt.

Cancer, Tumors, Leukemia, eye sight:

Grape/ seeds, apple seeds, peach seeds, apricot seeds, orange seeds, Garlic, cabbage, carrots, honey, lemon, oats, ginger, cauliflower, bitter kola, saw palmetto, soy, cocoanut/ oil, raisin, strawberry, spinach-(cataracts), bell pepper, kale(cataracts), broccoli, collard green, turnip green, see weeds, Brussels sprouts, endive(cataracts), water melon, oranges/seeds, cantaloupe, pawpaw, hot pepper, pumpkin seeds(prostrate and bladder problems), turmeric (cancer), dates, tangerine, cranberry (cancer/ tumors), avocado (oral / prostrate cancer, eye health), tomatoes, sunflower seeds (eye), salmon-omega 3

Tuberculosis:
banana cluster stem liquid, apricot seeds, bitter kola, oranges with seeds, peach with seeds

Anemia, tuberculosis, asthma, cough, bronchitis, respiratory health, pneumonia, Intestinal worms, Gallstones removal, Cleansing of Bile duct, Blood poisoning:
Apricot seeds, radishes, cucumber, red apple, grapefruits, honey, ginger, lemon, banana, Bitter Kola, lettuce, bell pepper, kale, collard green, mustard green, pineapple, water melon / seeds, oranges, cantaloupe, lime, pawpaw / seeds(expel worms), Cabbage, ginger, caffeine, lime, pawpaw leaves (relieves headache), sesame, turmeric (relieves pain), tangerine, sea salt

Spasm (sudden painful muscle contraction):Tangerine, sea salt.

Hair:
Lettuce and spinach (juice), okra wash, kiwi, lime, honey (conditioner).

Sores, eczema, leprosy, skin infections, leukemia, Diabetes, urinary tract infection, gastrointestinal ailments, digestion, constipation, colon health, worms, skin eruptions, chapped skin, burns, Swollen anal blood vessels (hemorrhoids), viral and bacterial infections (antibacterial), fungus(athlete's foot), High blood pressure reduction, blood circulation enhancer, colon cleanser, Body weight Loss, ulcer:

Bitter melon, Garlic, Okra, grapefruit, cabbage, cucumber, apple, honey, lemon, red onion, oats, ginger, cauliflower, banana, bitter kola, plantain (unripe),Grape/seeds, sea salt.

Saw palmetto, cocoanut & oil, raisin, broccoli (with honey,& ginger),lettuce, bell pepper, pineapple(warm repellant)/ digestion of protein, oranges, cantaloupe, lime, pawpaw / seeds (bleeding pile), pawpaw leaves(good for diabetes, purging, hernia, genitals), pepper (ulcer causing bacteria), bitter kola, alligator-pepper(antimicrobial), pumpkin seeds(intestinal parasites),Turmeric(eczema, ulcer, indigestion, anti—bacterial), pomegranate (blood thinning), dates(digestion, laxative), tangerine, cranberry, honey(antimicrobial, ulcer, wounds, sore), cranberry(anti bacterial, ulcer, urinary track health) ,cinnamon, sweet potato, dandelion vegetables (diabetes).

Malaria, Jaundice:
Bell pepper, oranges, lime, pawpaw,

Diphtheria, Sore throat:
Pineapple, lime, pawpaw (raw juice &honey on tonsils) or (Seasoned crushed ripe skin in vinegar)
Carrots, honey, cucumber, lemon, banana, grape / seeds and honey (sore throat with lime), sea salt.

Skin health, anti-wrinkle, anti-aging, acne, wart, skin horn, corn, Pimple, Skin growth, boil, freckles, ringworm, whitlow:
Grapefruit juice, grapefruit oil, cabbage, carrots, cucumbers, honey, lemon, Banana (anti-wrinkle: marsh and apply to face & wash off with cold water after 30 minutes), Grape/ seeds, cocoanut, kiwi, cantaloupe, lime, pawpaw latex/juice (helps boil & whitlow, horn, corn, pimple, dead skin cell cleanse,

smooth skin support), pawpaw (seeds paste for ringworm and latex for skin smoothness and disorder), tangerine, avocado (anti-aging), cranberry(body cleansing and urinary health), sea salt, almonds,

Blood Clot Prevention:
Pineapple.

High Blood Pressure Reduction:
Okra, celery, bell pepper, romaine lettuce, oranges, cantaloupe, lime, bitter melon, garlic, bitter kola, grapefruit, cabbage, cucumber, apple, honey, lemon, red onion, oats, ginger, cauliflower, banana, plantain(unripe),grapes with seeds, saw palmetto, coconut, raisin, broccoli (with honey and ginger), sea salt

Pineapple (warm repellant)/digestion of protein, oranges, cantaloupe, lime, pawpaw/seeds (bleeding pile), pawpaw leaves (good for diabetes, purging, hernia, genitals), hibiscus flower, tangerine, beets.

Thyroid Health:
Natural sea salt, see weeds, coconut / oil, pineapple,
Avocado, carrots, apricot, walnuts, sunflower seeds, fresh pepper,

Arthritis/Rheumatism, Gout, Varicose Vein (Inflammation of Veins):
Grapefruit, wheatgrass, fruit berries (cranberries, raspberries, blackberries, strawberries, blue berries), cucumber, apple, lemon, banana, grape/seeds, oranges, celery/(juice), Lemon, radishes, caffeine, bell pepper, mustard green, turnip green, Brussels sprouts, sea weeds, pineapple, water melon, cantaloupe, sesame, turmeric(arthritis, inflammation), pomegranate (osteoarthritis—cartilage damage prevention), tangerine,

Kidney, liver, gall bladder cleansing, hypertension reduction:

Spinach, parsley, lemon, banana, bitter kola, celery/juice, radishes, bell pepper, oranges, cantaloupe, pawpaw/latex/seeds (support liver), pumpkin seeds, hibiscus flower (liver, hypertension), turmeric, tangerine,

Refreshing air outside and inside the house:

Avocado plants

Remedies for Cuts, Wounds, burns, swelling, bruise:

Carrots, honey, cucumber, lemon, banana, banana-peel (for bruises) grapes with seeds, lime, pawpaw, turmeric (heals wounds), honey, sea salt.

Teeth, Gum, bone health/cleansing:

Apple, Soya, coconut, raisin, oranges, cantaloupe, sesame seeds, cram Berry (anti-plaque, bone health), cucumber, lime, lemon, strawberry.

Insect repellant:

Lemon peels.

Heartburn, digestion, constipation reduction of intestinal gas (carminative), diarrhea:

Lemon, ginger, Banana & sea salt (for, diarrhea, heartburn), Bitter Kola, bell pepper, pineapple, lime, turmeric, dates (for digestion, laxative), tangerine, cranberry (stomach),

Wasp, bee stings, mosquito bites to relieve pain:

Lemon, onion, banana peel, lime, pawpaw (papaya).

Stain remover, food preservative:
Lemon, lime.

Nervous system, Natural anti-depressant, memory health:
Oats, Grape seeds, saw palmetto, spinach, celery/juice, collard green, kale, turnip green, oranges, lime, turmeric (Alzheimer), multiple sclerosis (neuron sheath disorder),Dates (alcohol intoxication reduction)

Nausea prevention:
Ginger, pineapple, pawpaw, red palm oil,

Remedies for Urinary disorder:
Banana, cranberry (bladder/urinary track health), saw palmetto,

Allergies prevention:
Banana, honey.

Poison Ivy effect remedy:
Banana peel (rub inside peel on the rashes)

Measles and mumps remedy:
Bitter Kola and honey

Weight loss aids:
Okra, grapefruit, honey, cocoanut & oil, caffeine, celery/juice, bell pepper, cantaloupe, pepper, turmeric (metabolism), tangerine, avocado, walnuts, sea salt,

Reproductive health aids:
Unripe Plantain, honey, celery/juice, water melon, dates,

Menstrual disorder remedy:
Pawpaw (unripe), carrots juice,

Beverages (for good health):
Hibiscus flower (tea, soft drink), turmeric (+tea), pomegranate (juice), red cabbage drink,

Menopause relief:
Sea weeds, mustard green

Birth defect prevention:
Sea weeds.

CHAPTER 6

My Skin Care With food plants and the Believed cares:
Lemon, Lime, Cucumber, Almond etc.

Preparation for facial spray:
Crush lemon, lime, cucumber and almond,
Heat at low temperature and turn off heat before boiling point, sieve to filter out the liquid, after cooling, put the liquid in a spray bottle and spray on the face after shower morning and evening. Close the eyes as you spray. If you are allergic to the food plants, avoid these.
They can also be ingested. I have personally tried these and they work.

LEMON AND LIME
Reduces acne, eczema, rashes, bruises, removal of dead skin, dandruff (of the scalp), Shines the skin, disinfects, fights infection, removes odor,

CUCUMBER:
Reduces Swelling around the eye, deals with skin problems, Smoothens the skin

ALMOND:
Protects the skin with High vitamin E against U.V

Thoughts about watching what I apply on my skin developed after my health recovery experience with plants food regimen. I became more conscious of skin absorption and health effects of artificial ingredients in most cosmetics. That led to my adoption of food plants ingredients in my home made body care products. I started avoiding body care products with synthetic or artificial ingredients; to prevent skin absorption of toxins (artificial preservatives and color).

Epilogue

Natural health support from common food

Health is individual's responsibility and comes from common sense and discipline about what we eat and drink. Natural foods are better accepted by our bodies than processed foods. It is always good to see if home remedy could reduce or remedy our everyday problems before spending money on expensive medical treatments. We should also accept plant foods as our first healing remedy. The best is to form the habit of consuming food plants daily while you control or minimize the quantity of meat consumption. Fruits, nuts and vegetables are excellent natural support. They can remedy most of our common health problems.

Herbal medicine is the use of botanical remedies to support illnesses alleviation. Treatment of disease with plants has been around since ancient times. It has been used by all ancient societies of the world and it is still popular and effective till the present time. In most cultures where certain plant foods have been identified to prevent different types of diseases, the people adopt such foods as their natural health insurance and consume them as their staple foods. Medicinal foods when consumed as staple foods in certain cultures form the basis of traditional diets. People who know the value of natural foods from plants, take it as their responsibilities to eat variety of fruits, vegetables, nuts, consume considerably less animal foods and processed foods rarely develop ill health.

Herbalists generally like my grandfather believe that the body is a self-healing organism and that herbs should be chosen to enhance wellness. Enhancement of wellness prevents illness from gaining grounds in the human body. The human body is already created with various natural body chemicals and nutrients; lack of any, results to ill health. It is those natural agents from herbs that can help the body keep recreating itself. Any one who adopts the foregoing motto as a guiding principle for recreating the body would rarely get sick—**"More plant foods, less animal and processed foods" OR "More alkalizing foods and less acidifying foods."** Alkalizing foods help to keep off cancer which tends to thrive in acidified body cells.

The problem with processed foods is in the added ingredients and denaturing of foods in some processing. The body is healthier with natural plant foods. Some human bodies react to some additives, preservatives and coloring and some don't, depending on individuals' body chemistry.

My Grandfather's method of treating people was to first detoxify the body with certain plant root that purges; increase the patients consumption of alkalizing foods(fresh fruits, plant seeds, vegetables, and extracts from certain plant roots and tree barks) and decrease consumption of acidifying foods(animal foods, processed foods and drinks). Increase drinking of clean water.

I now consume a lot of vegetables and variety of fruits to balance and immunize my system with a lot of antioxidants.

Vegetables, fruits and seeds have numerous health benefits. Diets composed of more vegetables can constantly recreate your body, reduce the risk of chronic diseases, reverse aging and make you look 12 or more years younger than your chronological age.

Vegetables can supply the body with necessary nutrients like vitamins, minerals, and fiber that are vital for development and maintenance of the internal organs of the body. In addition, many vegetables contain disease-fighting natural medicine that can help reduce the risk of different kinds of cancer, heart disease, high blood pressure, diabetes etc.

All fruits and vegetables have each a set of its vitamins, minerals, antioxidants and other nutrients more specific to certain health support. From what worked for me, it is recommended that every one consumes on regular basis fruits and vegetables to reinforce the immune system and enable the body heal its self, prevent and reduce illnesses.

None Strenuous Exercise

I have continued with none strenuous elementary type of exercise for added metabolism and fitness of my body. Many elementary schools in different parts of the world still do the morning exercise and parade in the fields before the classes start. In some board schools of the world, evening exercise for the children is compulsory as part of children's health development. The benefits for the early morning exercise is for the sun's energy for good health; increase of the metabolic rate of the body which in turn energizes the body and gives the needed mental alertness. Do not strain or over do any exercise including weight lifting to avoid injuries that may lead to later life problems of arthritis. It is important to know your limits when doing any exercise. **I'm glad I got my life back after learning my lessons the hard way. You need not suffer first as I did before you can learn and hold on to the natural maintenance your body needs to prevent or reduce illnesses before they get bad.**

As it worked for me, it will work for you. You too can get your life back and be the first to take responsibility of your body and adhere to:

Geneses 1:29 **Then God said, "I give you every seed-bearing plant on the face of the whole earth and every tree that has fruit with seeds in it. They will be yours for food."**

Exodus 23:25 **"Worship the LORD your God, and his blessing will be on your food and water. I will take away sickness from among you,"**

Ezek. 4:9 **"Now take some wheat, barley, beans, peas, millet and spelt; Mix them all together an make bread"**

Sickness Prevention Summary:

A)Fresh air (oxygen): Saturate blood with oxygen by practicing breathing exercise. Adopt occasional none strenuous exercise to trigger metabolism and enhance normal breathing. Minimize shallow breathing. Allow fresh air into the rooms.

B) Toxins: Minimize consumption of toxins (synthetic or artificially flavored foods, preservatives and colors) and their application on the skin from body care products. Adopt safety precautions for the air you breathe. Wear mask if necessary in air polluted environment. Prevent inhaling toxins to the lungs.

C) Stress: Reduce stress and anxieties. Maintain positive attitude regardless of any adverse moment.

D) Acidifying foods: Reduce consumption of acidifying foods: example-Animal foods, dairy products, pop (artificial soft drinks etc), to prevent cancer; minimize or prevent blood cloth, stroke, heart attack, hardening of arteries, high blood pressure from:

-bad cholesterol (LDL) /plaques in the arteries;
-triglyceride (fat in the blood),
-homocysteine (toxic waste from digestion of protein-rich-food.)

E) Alkalizing foods: Create alkaline condition in the body by eating alkalizing foods from plants (fresh vegetables, fruits and nuts). Consume moderately, protein, carbohydrate and good fat (from plants) according to one's daily requirements. Drink enough clean water daily.

PH (potential of hydrogen): PH is a measure of acidity or alkalinity in the body cells. The scale ranges from 1to14 with 1 being very acidic, 7 neutral and 14 very alkaline. The ideal PH level for the body cells is around 7.2 to 7.35, just a little away from neutrality to a little on the side of alkalinity. Ideal body PH reduces and prevents ill health; while too much acid in the body cells promotes health problems including cancer. My experience got me convinced. PH testing paper strips as already mentioned are found at natural herb or health stores. PH can be checked from the saliva or urine first thing in the morning before breakfast.

F) Blood type diet[*]**:** Knowing one's blood type (A, B, AB, or O) helps one to set up food regimen compatible with one's blood type. It helps to improve digestion, avoid bloating or gas, constipation, lactose problem, allergy, heart disease, high blood pressure, cancer, and other illnesses, maintain healthy body weight, and live a healthier life.

G) Electromagnetic Radiation: Minimize exposure to electromagnetic radiation from lap tops, TV, cell phones etc. by adopting necessary precautions.

H) High Blood Sugar problem:
I observed that each time I ate large quantity of vegetables and small protein food like salmon and sardine fish for dinner; I got excellent glucose test result the following morning. I learned to minimize carbohydrate foods and drinks with sugar in the evenings. I rather consume more vegetables and small protein food in the evening to avoid high blood sugar problem the next morning. I learned to eat my supper early between 6.30-7pm. That gives the body enough time to process the food before bed time.

---

* Blood type diet:
"Eat Right 4 Your Type", D'Adamo states
en.wikipedia.org/wiki/Blood_type_diet
http://www.dadamo.com/video_intro.htm

Acknowledgements

My daughters, Dr. Sochi and Cheta, the Pharmacist and the Bio-Chemist who respectively encouraged me to write and share my testimony and my lessons to promote sickness prevention and natural cures, world wide,

My son Ifesi an Engineer, whose expertise in information technology inspired me on modes of publication. My second son Dilinna the planner fondly referred to as Organizer and my youngest son Chino the Economist all of who had been my esprit de corps boosters.

My wife Obiageli, an Administrator/Nutritionist, whose efforts to enforce consumption of food plants in our nuclear family had a passive impact on me.

Dr. Kwaku A. Appau (N.D), the Naturopath whose occasional interactions with me helped me recall the memories of my late grandfather's concepts of herbal remedies. He in some degree helped to edit the first print.

Endnotes

1. Grape Seeds: source-
American Association for Cancer ResearchOriginal article:
Ning Gao, Amit Budhraja, Senping Cheng, Hua Yao, Zhuo
Zhang and Xianglin ShiClinical Cancer Research, 15:
140-149, January 1, 2009
http://www.dietaryfiberfood.com/fruits-vegetables/ grape-seed-
extract-leukemia.php
http://www.oohoi.com/natural%20remedy/everyday_food/

2. Apricot:
A case-control study, published by the *Asia Pacific
Journal of Clinical Nutrition,* involved 130 prostate cancer
patients and 274 hospital controls.
http://apricotfacts.com/apricots/Health+Benefits+of+Apricots/

3. Garlic:
FASEB Journal 13(4): Abstract 209.12. en.wikipedia.org/wiki/
Garlic
http://www.desigram.com/Health/Ingredients/Garlic.html
http://www.oohoi.com/natural%20remedy/everyday_food/

4.Okra:
Junji Takano is a Japanese health researcher
Involved in investigating the cause of many dreadful diseases.
http://www.pyroenergen.com/articles07/okra-health-benefits.htm

5. Spinach:
Webmed
*http://www.webmd.com/eye-health/news/20041203/
eat-spinach-* prevent-cataracts

http://www.oohoi.com/natural%20remedy/everyday_food/

6. Turmeric: Health diaries
http://www.healthdiaries.com/eatthis/20-health-benefits-
of-turmeric.html
Nutritional supplement health guide:
http://www.nutritional-supplements-health-guide.com/
benefits-of-turmeric.html
http://www.oohoi.com/natural%20remedy/everyday_food/

7. Avocado:
Health Benefits of Avocado by: Junji Takan
http://www.pyroenergen.com/articles07/avocado-health-
benefits.htm
http://www.oohoi.com/natural%20remedy/everyday_food/

*8. Benefits of a Variety of Fruits and Vegetables
http://www.buildingbodies.ca/Nutrition/fruits-vegetables.shtml
RESOURCE BOX: Jane Oelke, N.D., Ph.D. is a
Traditiona l Naturopath and Doctor of Homeopathy in
southwest Michigan.
She is the author of Natural Choices for
Fibromyalgia" and "Natural Choices for Attention Deficit
Disorder.
She is a professional speaker on natural health topics. She can
be contacted at DoctorOelke@aol.com or through her website
at *www.NaturalChoicesForYou.com*
You can also read this article about *good diet plans* and what
a good healthy diet would look like.

9. Strawberry:
Health benefits of strawberry
Health & Beyond Online
http://chetday.com/benefitofstrawberry.htm

Strawberries Health Benefits
By *Bhakti Satalkar*
http://www.buzzle.com/articles/strawberries-health-benefits.html

*10. Researchers: More fruits, vegetables could reduce risk of stroke
Nation's Restaurant News, March 6, 2006
*http://findarticles.com/p/articles/mi_m3190/is_10_*
40/ai_n26692728/

11. Sea salt:
Living without drugs by Richard Sear
Natural Sea salt will not cause high blood pressure
http://www.natural-cancer-cures.com/natural-sea-salt.html
http://www.oohoi.com/natural%20remedy/everyday_food/

*12. Aspartame, MSG, and food colorings:
By sweetpoison.com
http://www.sweetpoison.com/ph-balance.html

13 . PH:
Balancing Acid/ Alkaline foods
http://www.trans4mind.com/nutrition/pH.html

14. Beets:
Daily Glass Of Beet Juice Can Beat High Blood Pressure, Study Shows
By science daily
http://www.sciencedaily.com/releases/2008/02/080205123825.htm

15. Bitter Kola:
Health benefits of bitter Kola
http://bittercolaworld.blogspot.com/2008/04/health-benefits- of-bitter-kola.html

16. Blood type diet:
"Eat Right 4 Your Type", D'Adamo states en.wikipedia.org/ wiki/Blood_type_diet
http://www.dadamo.com/video_intro.htm

17.Lemon: oohoi
http://www.oohoi.com/natural%20remedy/everyday_food/

18. Cabbage: ibid

19. Carrots: ibid

20. Celery: ibid

21. Cucumber; ibid

22. G rape fruit: ibid

23. Red onions: ibid

24. Cranberries: ibid

25. Turmeric: ibid

26. Banana: ibid "

27. Banana Stem extract
*http://www.best-home-remedies.com/herbal_* medicine/fruits/
banana.htm

28. Bible passages
NIV (New International Version) Bible.
http://www.biblegateway.com/passage/?search

29. Sleep: RUWC
http://www.restoreunity.org/sleep.htm

Note: * = wide coverage

www.ingramcontent.com/pod-product-compliance
Lightning Source LLC
Chambersburg PA
CBHW050335290526
45785CB00006B/2510